DEATH BY RHEUMATOID ARTHRITIS

CARLA JONES

DEATH BY RHEUMATOID ARTHRITIS

Published by Kindle Direct Publishing

Copyright © original 2010 and reprint 2020 by Carla Jones. All rights reserved.

Book cover art of Celia Veno, copyright ©2010, 2020 by Laura Gelsomini. Used with permission. All rights reserved.

All photos of Carla Jones and Celia Veno, copyright ©2010, 2020 by Carla Jones. All rights reserved.

All rights reserved. No part of this work may be used or reproduced in any form or by any electronic or mechanic means, without written permission from the author, except in the case of brief quotations embodied in critical articles and reviews.

CONTENTS

ACKNOWLEDGMENTS

INTRODUCTION

MY MOTHER **1**
THE DIAGNOSIS **8**
SIGNS AND SYMPTOMS OF SPINAL INSTABILITY **17**
TESTS THAT MAY BE ORDERED **17**
WHAT IS RHEUMATOID ARTHRITIS? **18**
THE CAUSE **19**
WHO IS SUSCEPTIBLE TO RA? **20**
MORTALITY/COMPLICATIONS FROM RA **21**

ACKNOWLEDGMENTS

As you may expect, this book is dedicated to my life example, best friend and Mother, Celia Veno. A friend and mentor, she guided me through this life with unconditional love, support, and prayers. Daily, I miss her peaceful presence and thoughtful ways. There are no adequate words to truly express everything my Mother meant to me.

I dedicate this book to my family. I value them and am grateful for their love and support.

This story is also dedicated to all who struggle daily with the pain and unknown fate that rheumatoid arthritis can threaten them with. My advice is, act to prevent the possible deadly outcome. Let early interventions and independent medical research act as your guide.

I thank God for blessing me with the privilege and opportunity to communicate my mother's story to the public. His daily regeneration keeps and revives me.

Many thanks to the host of individuals, that aided in the completion of this endeavor: Kayleigh Harris at Elsevier, Doug Kaufmann, Dr. Kristin Ingraham D.O., Dr. Andrea Marx, M.D., F.A.C.R., W. Hayes Wilson, M.D., Laura Gelsomini, and Dee Gould.

A special thank you is due to Karen Syed. Your kindness, patience, and guidance have been invaluable to me. The role you have played in this project cannot be understated. You have opened the door for me to shed light, on this overlooked tragedy.

INTRODUCTION

The intent of writing this book is to bring awareness to the fact that people can and have died from complications, due to rheumatoid arthritis. I experienced this reality firsthand. I lost one of my closest family members to the disease - my Mother. Rheumatoid arthritis eroded the vertebra of her cervical spine. This deterioration resulted in spinal cord syndrome. If my sister and I hadn't investigated her unusual symptoms full circle, we wouldn't have had any idea how she died; thankfully, we did. My account chronicles her medical and personal journey as she valiantly and gracefully fought RA. It also highlights potential deadly ties with the disease.

My hope and prayer are that the information in my story will save at least one person from dying such an excruciatingly painful and unnecessary death.

As I worked on medical research for this book I discovered, not one major media outlet covered the deadly complications that rheumatoid arthritis can bring. Perhaps it's fear. The fear of alarming those with RA that they should have even more to be concerned with than dealing with continual, lifelong pain, and complete immobility. If I were diagnosed with any disease, I'd want to be completely informed of the complications associated with the condition.

MY MOTHER

Digging through all my paperwork after she had died, I needed to find it. Social Security needed to know the cause of her death. After wading through old cell phone bills and greeting cards, there it was. Tucked in a yellow manila envelope, I found her Death Certificate. I knew what she died from, but it was still strangely confusing. Were they looking for something more technical? Opening it carefully, I read Celia Veno's death certificate, "Cause of Death: Rheumatoid Arthritis" She died from complications, due to arthritis that deteriorated her cervical spine, causing irreversible spinal cord damage.

Celia Veno was my mother and my best friend. The kind of mother every child dreams of having - loving, kind, encouraging, and gentle. Exceptionally calm with a disarming smile, the medium built brunette of Ukrainian lineage had a graceful demeanor and a quiet tolerance for the adversity's life would hand her. Being a content person, she was extraordinarily selfless and giving.

Life had not been easy for my mother, a daughter to a family of 10. Her father, Stanley, left his poverty-stricken home in the Ukraine region, in 1921 for the promised land of America. His hometown, the city of Kiev was then a founding republic of The Soviet Union. Ironically, her mother Veronica was on the same ship. Shortly after meeting, they fell in love. Two weeks later, they married.

This tall, lean, strong man with milky blue eyes would land in Olean, New York, and find a job as a laborer in a poisoned, air-polluted glass plant moving lime from boxcars to the warehouse. In the process, he withstood unendurable lime dust, a destroyer of lung tissues, and a breeder of silicosis.

Stanley and Veronica were quiet, loving, mild-mannered parents. They weren't given to yelling and cursing. They were a happy bunch, older children helped care for the younger siblings. During balmy summers, Mom would sit on her father's lap while he read The Olean Times Herald newspaper. Children scattered about, playing in the yard, dancing in the sunlight.

For her daughters, Veronica would hand weave together clover crowns made of the flower and a few spare bobby pins. Neatly she'd tuck the small crown ends behind the girls' ears. This family ritual of "crown-making" would be emulated by generations yet to come.

Following her back to the kitchen, the brood watched as she whipped up homemade bread and fresh galumpkis. A dish composed of cabbage leaves filled with fried beef, bacon, and rice, smothered in tomato sauce.

Weekly, the large-framed, jovial Veronica would set out on her usual bus ride to the downtown shops of Olean. She'd return with groceries and a small brown paper bag. As she approached the home, all those little eyes locked onto the smaller bag, knowing its all too familiar contents - candy. The children would sample the goods - licorice, and assorted hard candies.

While a man yet in his fifties, Stanley became tired and his bones began to ache. The doctor sat him down to tell him his diagnosis; the most aggressive type of arthritis - rheumatoid. That combined with his lungs wheezing from silicosis did not stop him from working. Bills had to be paid and a family to feed drove him on. He worked until he became crippled, unable to walk. In his early sixties, he was confined to a county nursing home. Quietly, he endured, crying out frequently of the pain that ran through his aching body. The drug of choice for rheumatoid arthritis in the 1960s was aspirin. At the time, some patients received twenty aspirin a day. This was the best doctors had to offer, knowing so little about the disease. Soon, his beloved Veronica was diagnosed with heart disease and high blood sugar. In their suffering, they eventually shared a room at the nursing home.

While at work, the hospital called my mother. It was an unexpected call. Her mother's heart burst from a fatal heart attack. Her father remained remorsefully alone. With his strength drained from years of relentless, crippling arthritis, Stanley, died only months later from a heart attack as well.

Letters were found later, from a village outside of Kiev from her father's sister. The two kept in touch and Mom paid a translator to help her read the Russian written letters. She was told her great-uncle was crippled and had a hard time walking. Perhaps he had rheumatoid arthritis, my mother thought. He is never mentioned again in her aunt's letters. Out of her nine siblings, my mother was the only one diagnosed with RA.

Growing up in the same small town and both having large families, my parents would hear of the other's family mentioned throughout the years. Even so, the two never met. Once, my mother remembered walking down the street near her home as a neighborhood boy caught her eye. He played with his dog by the sidewalk. As he looked into her eyes for a brief moment, she thought he must have gone to her school, but he was a new face to her.

With a quick passing, she gave no more thought to this boy and his dog. What she didn't know was that the two schoolmates would cross paths, at another time and in another place.

At twenty-one years of age, with her intensive blue eyes, flawless skin, pinned up, dark brown hair, and long legs, she was a vision of beauty. With her signature attire of black and white, she was quite eye-catching. However, having a splendid sense of fashion was only one dimension of the woman. She was an attentive listener, loyal, and kind to all. Blessed with a plethora of positive traits, she naturally attracted many friends.

A part of the social networking of the 1950s was gathering at restaurants or drugstores for a milkshake and burger. A small group of Mom and her friends went out one frigid night for such an outing. In February of 1952, they drove to a neighboring town in Portville, New York deciding on Red and Trudy's Restaurant. Driving up, the girls donning their A-line skirts and bobby socks, the friends made their way through the large snow-covered ground that had fallen over the last few days.

While gazing over the menu, one of her friends spied a group of peers she had known, sitting in another booth. One of Mom's mutual friends walked over and introduced the two. Standing before her was the nameless neighborhood boy of her youth. With wavy jet-black hair, he had transformed into a brawny, appealing young man. After sitting together and talking throughout the night, it was time for the gang to drive back to Olean. Dad volunteered to drive Mom home and before he dropped her off, he asked for her phone number. Without hesitation, she clearly penned it down. He called her the next day.

After a few years of courtship, the two married in 1957. The couple moved in with my father's parents, who lived in the same town. At that time, Mom began working at a department store called, Kitner's in Olean. Here her artistic talents were recognized and demonstrated, as she worked as a cosmetic consultant, selling for various lines. The brunette with cream-colored skin and a slim, shapely figure posed a striking sight behind the cosmetic counter. With a warm inviting personality, customers would flock to her for advice. Fervently, she enjoyed serving others in her family so, working with the public was an easy transition for her. Sent into New York City by her company, she attended several cosmetic schools. Classic companies as Faberge and Charles of the Ritz certified her as a consultant. Blending the perfect color for every skin tone, learning how to accompany dress color with eyeshadow, there was much to know. She excelled in her field.

In 1964, they had their first daughter, my sister. Dad worked at many different jobs. He and a childhood friend co-owned a barbershop and while working there, he thought daily of changing careers and becoming a writer. Knowing of this ambition, a mutual friend of my parents phoned him from Orlando, Florida, inquiring if he'd consider a position as a sportswriter for the Orlando Sentinel, a local newspaper. Talking it over with her, the two moved to Cocoa Beach, Florida in 1967. Later that year, he received another job offer, but this time it was for a newspaper, in Yonkers, New York. Without hesitation, my mother supported him and off they went to live in Dobbs Ferry, a New York City suburb.

Shortly after arriving there, I was born in North Tarrytown. The newer modest two-bedroom apartment was on the second floor and the tree-lined neighborhood was well kept. In 1971, a newspaper strike took my dad to Quakertown, Pennsylvania. He was named editor of a small county newspaper and we bought a newly built house. My parents looked forward to raising a family in that quiet farming community. They'd finally found our resting place.

After my sister and I went off to elementary school, Mom became employed as a sales and beauty consultant for Hess's Department Store and later worked for Merle Norman Cosmetics. Gathering all the tools of the trade, Mom would, "doll us up" as she liked to say, for school dances. While other girl's parents forbid them to wear makeup until they were older, our mom encouraged it.

"Foundation protects your skin. Oh, a little eyeshadow and lip-gloss won't hurt you" she'd whisper.

Applying and blending with a feather touch, she kept it natural and light. Happily, she passed her cosmetic knowledge on to her daughters and female friends.

In 1977, my father decided the two should separate and divorce. For many reasons, this devastated my mother. First, she loved him. In her heart, he was her soul mate, her life partner. Secondly, she was a mom with two young girls not knowing where to turn for support. Her closest family was five hours away in Western New York. She needed encouragement and had made friends but required more to help her through this crisis.

Having made a promise to her father-in-law, Louis, the two of them would drop my sister and me off at a local church every Sunday morning. The pair chose not to attend a place of worship for many years but continued to take us to church out of respect for my grandfather. I believe Divine Knowledge saw to it that the parsonage of that church sat directly across the street from our home. Many nights, the pastor and his wife would comfort and counsel my hurting Mother. Thoughts of God hadn't entered her mind so strongly after these sessions and she hadn't earnestly thought of Him since she was a teenager, she would recount. As she sat in a car on the beach, she wondered what life was all about, as we all have done, questioning her own existence. The pastor and his wife asked her if she would like to begin a new life by starting a personal relationship with God. They explained that through His Son there is hope, forgiveness, and eternal life. Desperate for some emotional relief, she said a simple prayer with the two.

After this short request, she instantly felt a peace she'd never known existed. She still suffered the pain of the divorce, but the bitterness toward my father had left her and she was able to forgive. The steady source of her strength and comfort now came from her unwavering faith in God. From this point on, she would share her new reason for hope with many.

After her conversion, she began attending church with my sister and me, and her relationship with my father improved greatly. The two eventually became good friends. Now her goal was to live the life that God had intended her to live, come what may.

Financially, she struggled down this new road of single parenthood. With two children to support, she needed to work full-time hours. In 1980, she accepted a job at a new retail store in town. Quickly, she learned many departments within the store and through the years garnered numerous awards for her outstanding work in customer service.

My father was supportive, continually helping her in every way he could. Despite just having enough to make ends meet, she was consistently generous with others and she would give a tenth of her income to our church. Whenever she had a little extra money, she'd surprise my sister and me with gifts, and support a multitude of charities. From the Fire Fighters to the Humane Society to World Vision, she felt compelled to help those less fortunate than her.

THE DIAGNOSIS

At fifty-eight, my mother had the beginning of what would be the biggest battle of her life. In the spring of 1984, her hands and feet began to ache, especially in the morning. The smallest outing would tire her, drain her, and even going to the grocery store was exhausting. Her general doctor wrote a prescription for blood work to investigate the problem. Her worst fear had been realized. She was diagnosed with rheumatoid arthritis. Her faith and positive attitude prevented her from wallowing in self-pity. Frequently she'd say, "Just remember, there's always someone out there who has it worse than you."

Her rheumatologist treated her with many different medications. First, she tried gold shots, then Prednisone and Ibuprofen; however, they offered only temporary relief from a life-dominating medical condition. Many times, she'd be consumed by numbing pain in her hands, arms, legs, and feet. Eventually, the extreme discomfort became intolerable. Slowly, through the years, her immunity to the painkillers would escalate. The doctor later prescribed Methotrexate, Imuran. Neurontin, and much-needed painkillers such as Darvocet. In 1995, a new narcotic hit the market, OxyContin. This strong painkiller brought a better comfort level to her, but its unexpected side effects would later come into play.

In the summer of 2003, her disease became so disabling; she needed to use a walker. The phone rang, and it was Mom. Her voice held a sense of urgency, "I think I twisted my ankle. I can't walk.", she said.

A decision to have her stay with my husband and I was immediately made. Visiting nurses, therapists, and nursing aids attended her. Mom made the best of it with her cheerful attitude. We were happy to have her, and she especially enjoyed playing with her seven-month-old grandson. We had asked her many times to come live with us. Thanking us each time, she declined, stating she didn't want to lose her independence.

We noticed that Mom slept most of the time and thought at first that the extra sleeping was brought on by depression. One afternoon, I sat and spoke with Mom and it was as if she was looking right through me, just staring off into the distance. Something was wrong. We'd noticed that she'd barely drunk any liquids the last two days, so we immediately called visiting nurses. The nurse explained that lack of fluids, combined with the Oxycontin, was causing her to become dehydrated, which made her disoriented. Concerned, my father arrived to help, and we took her to the emergency room.

While recuperating, from her dehydration, the doctor found a bone infection in her heel. Now she would need an operation and rehabilitation. After her surgery, she went to a rehab center. She began physical therapy on her arms and legs and was soon sitting up in a chair, preparing to go home. While there, she contracted a staph infection from an unclean pic line and almost died in December of 2003. Unhappy with this terrible incident, my sister and I arranged for her to recuperate at a different rehabilitation center.

We kept in constant contact with the dietitian, physical therapy department, the nursing department, and her doctors. One specialist that was not involved was her rheumatologist. It had been at least two years since her last appointment with him. After a quick phone call, he told us Mom was "burnt out" on arthritis medication and treatments. The doctor said it was the worst case of arthritis he'd ever seen, and that she had run the medicine gamut. After an exam, he suggested that she remain on the steroids for her inflammation and continue with the painkillers.

Physical therapists would make their daily rounds, to her room. Try as she might, she could barely sit up in bed, and when she could, it was only for short stints. Lifting her arms for a simple range of motion exercise was almost impossible. The therapist thought maybe she wasn't trying hard enough.

As discouraging as the situation was, my self-effacing mother did not complain. With her weakened, penetrating eyes, she said to me, "Carla, let's keep praying that I can walk again". Still not fully understanding why she couldn't walk, we prayed daily for a miracle. The doctors suggested she had developed weak leg muscles, due to becoming immobile for such a long time.

Unrelated symptoms began to materialize. Strangely, her skin would become uncomfortably warm and then switch abruptly to ice cold. This oddity happened continually day and night. She began to experience migraine-like headaches. Doctors prescribed allergy medications and Tylenol. Nothing stopped the pain, not even larger doses of OxyContin. Occasionally, she needed oxygen; we were told it was due to her sleep apnea. Later, we would learn that all these symptoms were due to a menacing cause, yet undetected.

As time went on, she could no longer tolerate any type of physical therapy and was unable to sit up, due to the headaches. Her MRI and CAT scan came back normal. Her bone-scan showed that she had spinal stenosis, osteoarthritis, and a small fracture from a previous fall located in her C3 and C4 discs. People with RA are at increased risk for osteoarthritis and studies show that bone loss in RA may occur as a direct result of the disease.[1] Her spinal stenosis was due to her natural aging process.

In early November 2004, Mom began to have severe

neck pain. After a visit to the neurologist, he ordered a cervical spine x-ray of her upper spine and found that Mom's C1 and C2 discs in her spine were deteriorating and thus, causing the pain. The specialist reassured the family that it was not a life-threatening condition but, if her neck pain continued, Mom may want to have an operation to repair the discs. They prescribed larger doses of Tylenol and OxyContin.

It was difficult and painful to watch my mother cope with unbearable arthritic pain the majority of her life. However, when she started experiencing these extreme headaches and neck discomfort, it became exceptionally disconcerting for all of us.

After considering the results from the cervical spine x-ray, I knew we should seek a second opinion from another neurologist and get a fresh diagnosis from a different rheumatologist.

It was now May 2005 and I'd arranged to accompany Mom to the appointment with the second rheumatologist, working out of Lehigh Valley Hospital in Allentown, Pennsylvania. For fourteen years in a row, *U.S. News and World Report's Guide to America's Best Hospitals* had recognized this hospital as one of the best in the country. I felt confident that a doctor practicing there would give us additional insight into Mom's spinal condition. At this point, her hands were becoming so numb that she could no longer hold her phone and she could barely feed herself. The nursing staff explained that this was due to the progression of arthritis. After reading her cervical spine x-ray sent from the neurologist and the examination, the doctor became solemn.

First, he said her headaches were coming from her deteriorating cervical collar pressing on the base of her skull. Headaches originating in the cervical collar are called, "cervicogenic." When one experiences a cervicogenic headache, pain is felt in the head, but its source resides in the cervical spine. These types of headaches are caused by mechanical problems of the cervical spine. Vertebral arteries pass through the cervical vertebrae and any disruption would affect these arteries, possibly decrease the blood supply to the head, causing a headache. They are frequently confused with migraines.[2] He also found something imperative that the neurologist missed.

Looking into her eyes he said, "Your C1 and C2 are very badly damaged and your spine is compressing on top of itself. This is called spinal cord syndrome. You have the same thing that Christopher Reeve has. His C1 and C2 broke instantly when he was thrown off his horse. Your condition is progressive. It's as though there is a floating knife in your back. This knife consists of fragmented bone from your spine. From any small movement, this knife will cut off one or all of your bodily functions, such as your heart or your breathing. You'll die if you don't get an operation to get this repaired."

Disbelieving what we'd just heard, we both asked him, if her condition was truly fatal.

Quietly, he said, "Yes."

He said the operation would be risky because of the advancement of the damage to her spinal cord. Even so, he thought she held some hope of survival, for her heart and lungs were still healthy and strong, even at seventy-four years old.

For people with RA, the effects of arthritis on the spine can vary from minimal symptoms to life-threatening pressure on the spinal cord. This requires complicated surgery to stabilize the spine and reduce the pressure on the spinal cord. Spinal cord pressure can result in, numbness or weakness in the arms and fingers, pain in the neck and or arms, lack of coordination. Pressure on the vertebral arteries can lead to blackouts when the blood flows through these arteries is reduced, and the same thing occurs when you move your head and neck a certain way. When the joints of the spine are destroyed, the connection between each vertebra becomes unstable. The problem of joint instability is profoundly serious when it occurs between the C1 and C2 vertebrae in the cervical spine, for they control all of your life-sustaining functions.[3]

She would require a surgery called an anterior cervical discectomy, the most frequently used procedure to fix damaged cervical discs. After making a small incision in the front of the neck, the disc material pressing on the spinal nerve is then completely removed. The bone channel is enlarged, giving the nerve more room to exit the spinal canal. The open space is then filled with bone graft taken from the pelvic region. The slow process of the bone graft joining the vertebrae together is called "fusion." Spinal fusion is a surgery that combines two or more vertebrae. This procedure is used primarily to eliminate the pain caused by abnormal motion of the vertebrae.[4]

My mind was spinning with questions. Any time she moved she ran the risk of dying? What if *I* moved her the wrong way? What if a nurse or aid did? How did she get two different diagnoses from the same x-ray? Physical therapy was dangerous for her... After this devastating diagnosis, Hospice became involved with her treatment plan.

During one of our many visits, she said, "Don't worry; I'm going to see my baby girl." She was referring to her unborn granddaughter. During each one of my sister's and my pregnancies, Mom would lovingly pat our bellies, and jokingly say, "Little Cecelia's in there." (Cecelia was

Mom's birth name.) After one of my ultrasounds, I called her from the hospital's parking lot with news of her first granddaughter. Emotionally thrilled, through her tears, I heard her sweet, trademark laugh. "I'm so happy for you Carla." It was clear she was anticipating the upcoming arrival. I informed her of the baby's middle name – Cecelia.

Complications arose in my pregnancy and I became a gestational diabetic. Through my diabetes classes at the hospital, I learned there was a chance that my daughter could be born with significantly low blood sugar levels. If this was the case, she may need to have glucose administered by IV at birth.

Another risk would be an increase of insulin in her system and this could cause her to have breathing difficulties. As she was my best friend, I shared this unsettling news with my mother. Handling every problem with prayer, she put her hand on my stomach and asked God to bless my baby with health and no complications, and that she would not need any IVs. Suddenly, relief swept over me.

After a local neurologist examined Mom, he consented to operate, but shortly after changed his mind, stating he did not feel the outcome would be positive, due to the advanced stage of her condition. Her rheumatologist recommended Thomas Jefferson Hospital, in Philadelphia, and there we found an experienced neurosurgeon.

With her cervical spine being as fragile as an eggshell, moving her was nerve-wracking and frightening. The hour trip to Philadelphia was a nightmare, for during the ride Mom said she almost lost consciousness. I knew it was a risky decision, but it was the only way to save her. After talking to the neurologist at Thomas Jefferson, the prognosis did not look promising. His exact words were, "I wouldn't let someone do this operation on my mother. There is a 90% chance she will die during the operation." He went on to say that in order to get to the C1 and C2, they would have to go in through her mouth and there would be much blood loss. She would have to wear a brain halo for a year until she finally healed, and she would have a long recovery. He said that if she were diagnosed with spinal cord syndrome before it had progressed to this point, she would be a candidate for a successful surgery.

My mother opposed the surgery, knowing the risk that was involved. She stated, "I'm just going to trust The Lord."

As always, her hope in Jesus gave her assurance for whatever lay ahead.

When she returned from the hospital, it was apparent that her condition had worsened. With complete loss of movement of her body from the neck down, she now needed a special call bell to summon the nurses. It was a flexible microphone-looking piece, which was activated by the user blowing air, into its mouthpiece. After a few short days, her breathing worsened and the bell became useless. Hospice informed us that her body was shutting down. Her kidneys were no longer functioning, the first sign of decline.

My sister and I took turns around the clock sitting at her bedside. Upon learning of her worsening condition, my father cut a visit short in their hometown in New York driving all night to get back to Allentown, Pennsylvania. Without sleep, he stayed up that day and the entirety of the following night with her. Just the two of them quietly talking about family, friends, and other ties that bound their 55-year relationship.

The next day while I was at her side, she slept and then slipped away. Her struggle with chronic, unbearable pain was over. The date was July 19, 2005.

Thirty-eight days later, my daughter was born. She was perfectly healthy. All of her sugar-levels were normal, and she had no breathing problems.

Hospice workers, for the first time, requested to counsel a handful of nursing staff. They were the ones that cared for my Mother. She was one that had a genuine gift of compassion and empathy. Both traits worked as a magnet for those who knew her. Despite her many difficulties, she supported others in any way she could. Her remarkable qualities surfaced during her last weeks, as her time was spent requesting visitors, to leave soda tabs to raise money for infant defibrillators, benefiting a nearby hospital.

The Spine Journal notes that "Eighty-six percent of patients with rheumatoid arthritis, have cervical spine involvement. Often these lesions are clinically asymptomatic, and the symptoms are erroneously attributed to peripheral manifestations of the patient's rheumatoid disease. Because these lesions are common and missed diagnosis can result in death. Cervical spine involvement of RA is common and progressive. Early recognition is vital."[5]

Dr. Kristin Ingraham D.O., Assistant Professor of Clinical Medicine at Lehigh Valley Hospital, in Allentown, Pennsylvania recommends those falling into three categories need cervical spine x-rays.

"We require cervical spine x-rays for all patients before surgery, any patient with longstanding rheumatoid arthritis and for any patient with symptoms of headaches, neck pain, or numbness of arms and legs. What we look for on the x-ray is subluxation, which is the instability of the spine. Moreover, when there is instability, the spinal cord is in danger of becoming compressed. It's better to stabilize the spine before there are neurological problems. Any evidence of damage and the patient would need to go to a neurosurgeon for stabilization", Ingraham said.

She also added what action should be taken if extensive damage was found. "The rheumatologist calls the neurosurgeon if symptoms are extreme." The term for the spinal instability of the C1 and C2 is called "atlantoaxial subluxation." Dr. Ingraham's advice on those who have been diagnosed with RA in their spine: "Definitely get regular checkups by the rheumatologist to make sure there is no neurological damage and that there is no weakness in their arms or legs. Patients can request that a cervical spine x-ray is done if they are experiencing any symptoms."

SIGNS AND SYMPTOMS OF NECK INSTABILITY

- Weakness, paralysis
- Breathing difficulties (from paralysis of the breathing muscles)
- Spasticity (increased muscle tone)
- Sensory changes
- Numbness
- Pain
- Loss of normal bowel and bladder control (such as constipation, incontinence, bladder spasms)
- Blood pressure irregularities
- Abnormal sweating/trouble maintaining regular body temperature
- Migraine-like headaches.[6]

TESTS THAT MAY BE ORDERED

- Spine x-rays- may show fracture or damage to the bones of the spine.

- A CT (cervical spine x-ray) or MRI - may show the location and extent of the damage.
- Myelogram -an x-ray of the spine after injection of dye may be necessary in rare cases.
- Somatosensory Evoked Potential (SSEP) Testing - may show if nerve signals can pass through the spinal cord. [7]

WHAT IS RHEUMATOID ARTHRITIS?

(RA) is a chronic inflammatory autoimmune disorder that causes the immune system to attack the joints. It causes loss of mobility due to pain and causes joint destruction. It also affects the tissues throughout the body including the skin, blood vessels, heart, lungs, and muscles. The disease is also associated with depression.[8]

Joints become swollen, tender, and warm and their movement is limited by stiffness and pain, especially in the morning. Traditionally, the stiffness will last for more than one hour. Most frequently, the smaller joints are affected such as the hands, feet, and cervical spine. Larger joints such as the shoulder and knees can also be involved. The joints affected have a symmetrical pattern. (Both sides of the body are affected, example right and left knees) Warmth is felt around the affected joints. Rheumatoid nodules can be found on a smaller percentage of patients. These are lumps found under the hands and elbows. Fatigue, loss of energy, low-grade fevers, loss of appetite, and enema dry eyes are also hallmarks of the disease.[9]

It is diagnosed on symptoms and signs, but a blood test called "rheumatoid factor" is normally taken. Doctors look for certain antibodies linked to the disease. Oddly enough, 15% of those with a negative blood test have the disease. A rheumatologist who will treat and manage the disease performs diagnosis. Treatments include physical and occupational therapy, painkillers, steroids, and biologics. Biologics are new treatments that involve DNA and technology. Diseases modifying anti-rheumatic drugs are also used in treatment. These drugs are used to slow down the disease.[10]

THE CAUSE

The cause of rheumatoid arthritis is mysteriously unknown. Infections such as viral, bacterial, and fungal have been suspected but have yet to be proven. Doug Kaufmann noted author and speaker, sites fungus as the primary catalyst in many diseases, including RA. In his book, *The Fungus Link,* he includes medical research confirming the connection between arthritis and fungus. In the book, *The Townsend Letter for Doctors,* nineteen doctors wrote of a condition known as candidiasis (from the yeast Candida) and how it could mimic symptoms associated with RA. One of the authors, physician Dr. Costantinis, found evidence that mycotoxins (from fungi) caused RA. If one has not had success with their treatments, Doug Kaufmann recommends talking with your physician about prescribing any one of several systemic antifungal medicines for a few weeks. While taking the medication, he recommends a diet void of sugars, dairy products, peanuts, corn, and other fungi's related foods for a month or two. These are foods that he believes, feed fungi in the joints. He includes a "Phase I" diet in his book *The Fungus Link.* If this regiment works, Kaufmann suggests terminating the drugs and try herbal anti-fungal remedies.[11]

The tendency to develop RA may be genetically inherited. It is also suspected that certain infections or factors in the environment might trigger the activation of the immune system. One current theory is that a person who is genetically predisposed to RA encounters a trigger (an infection, virus or bacteria, or the environment). The trigger starts an abnormal immune response. More than one gene is involved in determining whether a person develops RA and how severe the disease will become. Scientists also believe that a variety of hormonal factors may be involved.[12]

WHO IS SUSCEPTIBLE TO RA?

Roughly 75% of all those diagnosed with RA are women. This suggests that genetics and hormones may play some role in the cause. The average age of those who are diagnosed is between 30 and 60 but any age, including children, can develop the disease. People of all races and backgrounds can develop RA Today an average of over 1.5 million people live with RA in the United States. [13]

MORTALITY/ COMPLICATIONS FROM RA

Rheumatoid arthritis has long been intertwined with high mortality. RA patients have had much higher rates than the overall population of heart disease, vascular disease, and congestive heart failure. Being linked with an increase in mortality and morbidity, there are varieties of potentially fatal medical conditions that are birthed by rheumatoid arthritis. Of those diagnosed with the disease, 15-25% will experience complications involving organs of the body such as the heart and lungs. One such connection is that of RA and cardiovascular deaths. Those with RA have significantly higher rates than the overall population of heart disease, vascular disease, congestive heart failure, and stroke. The reason being is that inflammation is a risk factor for cardiovascular patients and patients with RA represents a higher risk group because their disease involves inflammation.[14]

Lungs are also affected in some patients with RA. They can develop lung nodules, excess tissue in the lungs, and pleural effusion. Pleural effusion is an additional fluid that collects in the space surrounding the lungs. It can interfere with normal breathing by not allowing the lungs to expand properly during inhalation. Autopsies have shown that 40-70% of RA patients have a pleural disease. Respiratory infections account for 15-20% of deaths for those with RA.[15]

Dr. Hayes Wilson, Chief rheumatologist at Piedmont Hospital and medical advisor to The Arthritis Foundation in Atlanta calls RA a "very important and deadly disease." He went on to say, "It does not just take two aspirin and call me in the morning. Get an early diagnosis and treat it aggressively. The consequence of not treating it aggressively could be excess mortality. We need to find out why it's killing people."[16]

Currently, new methods for determining which patients are more likely to develop a more aggressive type of the disease, are becoming more readily available. Recent research has found that the presence of "citrulline antibodies" in the blood have been associated with a greater tendency toward more destructive forms of RA. Studies involving different types of connective tissue collagen are in progress and show encouraging signs of reducing rheumatoid disease. B cell depletion using the anti-CD20 antibody, rituximab, is shown to be an effective tool in treating RA.[17]

Diagnosed two months before she died, my mother could have had many more years to live. If the source of her symptoms were detected, six months to a year earlier, she would have been eligible for immediate corrective surgery that most likely, would have saved her life. If anyone you know has Rheumatoid Arthritis in their cervical spine, they need to stay connected to their rheumatologist and know the warning signs of spinal instability. A spinal cord injury is considered a medical emergency and requires immediate treatment to reduce long-term effects. Quadriplegia and or death can follow an injury if it is not caught promptly. Time is critical.

My readers become my fellow advocates, whenever necessary, empower those around you with *more* knowledge of this unpredictable disease called rheumatoid arthritis. You never know who you will interact with in life to share this information with. You may be a healthcare professional, treating a patient. Perhaps you're a physical therapist who hasn't considered cervical damage as a possible roadblock as to why your patient with RA just can't tolerate movement due to their headaches. You may be a parent of a child with RA, needing to ask the right questions about cervical degeneration at their next rheumatologist's appointment. You may be the one with RA and are starting to experience these seemingly unrelated symptoms.

Not only does rheumatoid arthritis have the capacity to take away your ability to function in your daily life, but it can also completely cripple you, steal your independence, and then eventually kill you. Don't ignore the warning signs. Don't avoid your rheumatologist and stop putting off that much recommend a spinal x-ray. It could be the last thing that you do.

WORKS CITED

[1] Medline Plus, A service of the U.S. National Library of Medicine and the National Institutes of Health: (Aug 3, 2009). Used with permission.

[2] Medline Plus, A service of the National Institute of Neurological Disorders and Stroke, U.S. Dept. of Health and Human Services. (Aug. 3, 2009). Used with permission.

[3] Medline Plus, A service of the National Institute of Neurological Disorders and Stroke, U.S. Dept. of Health and Human Services. (Aug. 3, 2009). Used with permission.

[4] The Free Dictionary by Farlex. (2004)

[5] This article was published in, *The Spine Journal* Vol. 4, Issue 6, (Nov-Dec 2008) Francis H. Shen MD, Dino Samartzis BS, Louis G Jenis MD, and Howard San. "Rheumatoid Arthritis Evaluation and Surgical Management of the Cervical Spine." Page 689 Copyright 2008, with permission from Elsevier.

[6] Medline Plus, Bethesda, (MD) A service of the U.S. National Library of Medicine and the National Institutes of Health, Spinal Cord Trauma (Jan 7, 2007). Used with permission.

[7] Medline Plus, Bethesda (MD) A service of the U.S. National Library of Medicine and the National Institutes of Health, Spinal Cord Trauma (2007). Used with permission.

[8] Medline Plus, Bethesda, (MD) A service of the U.S.

National Library of Medicine and the National Institute of Health, National Institute of Arthritis and Musculoskeletal and Skin Disease. (2007) NIH Publication # 09-4179. Used with permission.

[9] Medline Plus, Bethesda, (MD) A service of the U.S. National Library of Medicine and the National Institute of Health, National Institute of Arthritis and Musculoskeletal and Skin Disease. (2007) NIH Publication # 09-4179. Used with permission.

[10] Wikipedia – Rheumatoid Arthritis, Nishimurak Sugiyama D. Kogata Y, et al (2007 June) Ann. Intern Med 146 (11) p 797-808. Used with permission.

[11] Kaufmann, Doug, and Holland, David (2000), *The Fungus Link*, 1st edition, Media Triton Volume 1, 2nd series David Holland, MD *Arthritis The Fungi Connection* – p 35, 36, 37. Used with permission from Doug Kaufmann and David Holland, MD.

[12] National Institute of Arthritis and Musculoskeletal Skin Diseases – "Nature of Genetics", G Gegersen PK, Amos CI, Lee AT, Lu Y, Remmers EF, Kastner DL, Seldin MF, Criswell LA, Plenge RM, Holers Vm, Mikuls TR, SOkka T, Moreland LW, Bridges SL, Xie G, Begovich AB, Siminovitch KA, REL (June 7, 2009): 41-820-823. Publication #04-4179. Used with permission.

[13] Medline Plus, Bethesda, (MD) A service of the U.S. National Library of Medicine and the National Institute of Health, National Institute of Arthritis and Musculoskeletal and Skin Disease. (June 9, 2009) NIH Publication # 09-4179. Used with permission.

[14]This article was published in the, *RA Record*, Reprint from the Am J Med 121. Libby P. *Role of Inflammation in atherosclerosis associated with rheumatoid arthritis*, S21-S31. Copyright 2008, with permission from Elsevier.

[15] The Johns Hopkins Arthritis Center, Baltimore MD- Dr. Andrea Marx, *Pulmonary Involvement in Rheumatoid Arthritis*. John Hopkins Medicine, Baltimore, MD. JohSem Arthritis Rheum 24: 242-54, Copyright 1995, with permission from Dr. Andrea Marx.

[16] Wilson, Hayes, MD Chief of Rheumatology Piedmont Hospital, Atlanta, GA and Medical adviser, Arthritis Foundation, Atlanta, GA (Nov 2007)). *Journal of Arthritis & Rheumatism,* with permission from Hayes Wilson.

[17] "Genetic Markers of Treatment Response in Rheumatoid Arthritis", Vol 50, Issue 4, (April 2004) by S. Louis Bridges, page 1019-22, Copyright 2009, with permission from Elsevier.

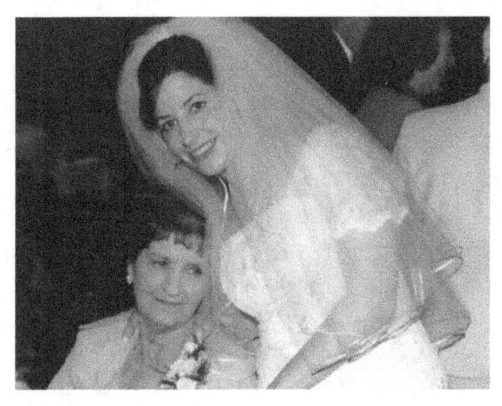

My Mom and I - 2000.

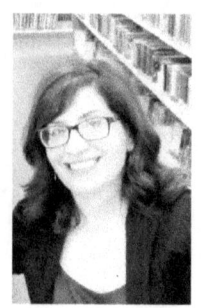

CARLA JONES has been writing professionally for twenty-plus years for various print and online publications including *The Morning Call Newspaper, Lehigh Valley Women's Magazine, The Country Register, and The Lehigh Valley Press.* She lives in Southeastern, Pennsylvania with her husband and children.

Mrs. Jones donates the entirety of her book royalties to the non-profit organization, the Rheumatoid Patient Foundation (rheum4us.org) established by her dear friend Kelly O'Neill Young aka "RA Warrior". The author is a proud Partner and Advisory Board Member for RPF. Kelly's organization is, "dedicated to improving the lives of those living with the disease" and their vision is to "envision a world where no one suffers from rheumatoid disease".

For additional information on the complexities and complications of rheumatoid disease, read Kelly's best-selling, comprehensive handbook, *Rheumatoid Arthritis Unmasked: 10 Dangers of Rheumatoid Disease.*

www.ingramcontent.com/pod-product-compliance
Lightning Source LLC
Chambersburg PA
CBHW070943220526
45469CB00007B/2501